## Table of Contents

The Heart ................................................................. 3

Public Health ........................................................... 6

Medications ............................................................. 9

What is the American Medical Association? ............... 11

Epidemiology .......................................................... 14

Heart Failure .......................................................... 17

Congestive Heart ................................................... 19

What is CHF? .......................................................... 21

Congestive Heart Failure ......................................... 24

CHF Diagnosis ........................................................ 26

**New Therapies for Treatment of CHF** ..................... 29

Top Hospitals- Lower Mortality Rate ........................ 32

Patients' Needs for a Healthy Heart ......................... 35

Combat Congestive Heart Failure ............................. 37

Saving the Heart .................................................... 40

Living With Heart Failure ......................................... 42

Current Research on CHF ......................................... 45

Peer Review in Medical Research ............................. 47

Treatment of Congestive Heart Failure ..................... 49

Translational Research ............................................ 53

Stem Cells Use in Congestive Heart Failure .............. 56

Genes Contribute to and Cure Congestive Heart Failure ........... 59

Continuing Medical Education .......................................62

Enjoy the Highest Quality of Life Possible With CHF .................65

Cardiac Professionals ...............................................68

# The Heart

The heart one of the most talked about part of your body. The heart used metaphorically describes love as well as a great hurt like broken heart. "My heart over flows with the love I have for you," says a young lover to his sweetheart. The emotions that we express with our heart are only part of the human makeup. The other part consists of having a healthy heart.

The heart is a real part of your body organs and functions to keep you alive and healthy. It is a noted fact that not only emotions affect your heart but also your food, your lifestyle, exercises, and stress all play a pertinent part in heart health. The American Heart Association provides much information about heart care. The Cleveland Clinic and other medical centers provide information and steps you can take to have a healthy heart.

Exercise is very import part of a healthy heart care. We know that not everyone can go to the gym or has the room in their home for gym equipment. We have some suggestions that will help your heart health.

- Set in a comfortable chair loosen your clothing for comfort.

- Start with your feet and ankles; rotate them so that you feel the strain.

- Work up to your legs raising them up and holding them for about five minutes.

- Work your hands and arms one side then the other.

- Next, work your head up and down then back and forth.

About 20 minutes a day will help you relieve stress in your life and let you relax. This is a good way to improve on heart health. The next thing is your diet plan remember it is not what you eat but how much and how often. We suggest you stay away from the normal things that people talk about like fats, too many sweets, and things that you know will harm you.

The heart is measured by taking your blood pressure with results letting your physician know your condition. When reading your heart first the doctor looks at the Systolic level because systolic heart failure occurs when the left ventricle cannot contract vigorously which is a pumping problem? The diastolic heart failure occurs when the left ventricle cannot relax or fill fully which becomes a filling problem. The heart must be able to pump vigorously and then relax to refill with blood to have a healthy heart.

AHA has put together some prime information and published it while the U.S. Government has not attempted to track heart disease. The AHA feels strongly that the government should get involved.

Yes, the heart is the soul of our existence. For many we think of the heart when we are in love or at a time of loss love. As we grow older then we venture to look at the real heart the arteries, veins, and the effects on our heart by the things we do. Take heart and enjoy your life.

# Public Health

Experts are outraged over the fact that the U.S. Government does not track Heart Diseases. American Heart Association feels that since heart failure is the number one killer amongst men and women that it should concern the government since it does concern the public health. Our government should track national rates of heart disease and stroke to help cut the incidences of these prime causes of death.

Currently data is collected by different sources and then published once a year in the AHA annual Heart Disease and Stroke Journal. The Public Health does not keep a record of heart diseases as they do for other illnesses. The doctors of today have to rely on information provided by different sources as journals and magazines. The Public Health is for everybody's concern and since the government controls this division, it is highly advisable that they start tracking patients with heart problems.

It is true that the American Heart Association has been doing a great job compiling this information from many and various sources. The fact is that there are many missing pieces, and it is not a good idea to have a nongovernmental agency, with no authority to modify data collected. The fact that the Public Health Department has no control over the facts or evaluation means that changes are slowly improved.

The Public Health Department has the capability of being a surveillance unit that can evaluate how data gets collected then make changes as needed. The Public Health Department can make sure that everyone in the medical field has access to all the information concerning the heart.

It is up to the Public Health Department to gather the needed information from the primary physicians, simply have the physicians report heart disease and stroke whenever possible. The information shared with doctors and patients would be much more obtainable. The public is under the false impression that the medical field is well informed about heart diseases. The truth about the situation is that there is no formal method of collecting data. That in reality without the efforts of the AHA doctors would not be as advanced as they are today concerning heart related problems. The current data collected by surveys needs some modification to help with increasing the physician's capability to treat heart patients.

- National surveys should expand existing questions on risk factors for heart disease, stroke, and other vascular diseases. Include in the survey risk factors such as physical inactivity, unhealthy diet, smoking and obesity.

- The Public Health System should standardize data collection across existing surveys to eliminate duplication and make information easier to compare.

- Laboratory results on cholesterol levels and blood sugar control to information collected from physician visits needs to be compiled for the possibility of discovering any connections to heart problems. The Public Health

Department duty should be to maintain these records for our own safety and well-being.

Let us note that heart health is of interest to the U.S. Food and Drug Administration offers advice on how to keep your heart healthy.

# Medications

Medications are important when it comes to healthy heart care. The patient needs to understand how the proper medication affects the heart. The fact that the heart has different problems means that accordingly the medication may vary as well. It is possible to have multiple problems such as high blood pressure and cholesterol then you would need two different types of medications.

The medicine that is Beta-Blockers, which reduce the heart rate and the output of blood by counteracting a hormone called noradrenalin, is not recommended for people with severe heart failure. Diuretics are a medication that helps people with fluid retention. The digitalis medicines increase the force of the heart's contractions, helping to improve circulation. The medicines known as Angiotensin converting enzyme (ACE) inhibitors and Angiotensin II receptor blockers (ARBS) may improve survival among heart failure patients and may slow or prevent the loss of heart pumping activity. The ACE inhibitors were originally developed as a treatment for high blood pressure the inhibitors help heart failure patients by decreasing the pressure inside the blood vessels. This results in the heart not needing to work as hard to pump blood through the vessels. Nitrate or hydralazine is prescribed to patients who cannot take ACE inhibitors or ARBS. These medications help relax tension in blood vessels and improve blood flow.

These are the basic groups of medications but they are manufactured by drug companies that attach their own name, however, just read the explanation you will get from your pharmacist and that will let you know the type of medication you are taking. Patients with high cholesterol levels take a drug called Lipitor while another patient might be in need of a Beta-Blocker so the medicine named Plavix. A patient might be inclined to strokes; therefore Nadolol helps with this problem. One medication that you can take that is highly recommended is Bayer Aspirin 81mg. The Aspirin known to stop heart attacks or prevent heart attacks and this medicine bought over the counter without a prescription.

The above medications are just a few that your doctor can prescribe for you according to your heart condition. The heart is one of the most vital organs in our body. It is essential that we take care of our heart in order to survive. That is why taking medications are a very serious matter. This could prevent your heart from functioning. I knew a man who was not of the wisest nature and whenever he traveled on his short weekend trips would take all of his heart medications on Friday afternoon so he would not have to take them with him. The first time he proclaimed that the room went round and he was dizzy for a while. This did not stop him the next time he did this when he stood up his heart stopped. Yes, the man died at the age of 55 years simply because he mismanaged his medications. Please only take what your doctor recommends and only as it is prescribed.

# What is the American Medical Association?

The AMA is an association of doctors that strives to further medical education and promote advancement of medical care for all persons. Ever since its foundation in 1847 at the University of Pennsylvania, the American Medical Association has had its hand in many of the major issues pertaining to medicine and medical research.

Perhaps the most widely known of the American Medical Association's accomplishments is the publication of JAMA, the Journal of the American Medical Association. Published forty eight of the fifty two weeks in a year, this peer reviewed scientific journal is the most widely circulated journal publication in the world. Here medical professionals can find information on all health related fields, including public health and advancement in underprivileged countries. They maintain a high level of excellence, rejecting ninety two percent of the articles submitted to them annually. This journal is made available at no cost to physicians in underdeveloped areas and is an invaluable source of continuing education for clinicians in any field.

The AMA has established a website, www.ama-assn.org which is a valuable tool to clinicians and patients alike. Here members of the AMA can follow current activities of the association, such as its actions in Washington with regards to the current Medicare controversy. The association has throughout history taken pride in its role in supporting or opposing legislation with regards to the medical community coming out of Washington.

A listing of continuing education opportunities has been listed, a vital tool as all health care professionals are required to complete a minimum number of continuing education credits per year. Information concerning HIPAA (the Health Insurance Portability and Accountability Act) can also be found here. This act dictates how physicians' offices should submit claims to third party payers such as insurance companies so as to best protect their patients' privacy and prevent personal medical information from becoming public knowledge, a delicate juggling act for many.

The association plays a major role in helping many students to enroll in and complete medical school. At www.ama-assn.org students are given access to a wide listing of possible careers in the medical field, as well as assistance in choosing a medical school and, following completion of their course of study, how to become licensed in their state of residency. Here students will also be able to obtain information on financial aid, perusing grants and scholarships made available through the AMA as well as advice on how to pay for college using funding not available through the association.

For non-physicians the AMA also provides a DoctorFinder on their website, a process by which patients can search listings of hundreds of doctors which are registered with the AMA to select the family physician, pediatrician or specialist that best fits their needs. The name, address and phone number is listed; some doctors may choose to place more information concerning themselves and their practice under their listing. All physicians registered with the AMA are required to be appropriately qualified to practice medicine in their chosen community, and must comply with the standards for ethics established by the association, making the AMA DoctorFinder an invaluable tool when a patient must search for a physician in an area with which they are unfamiliar.

# Epidemiology

Epidemiology is the process of where one is able to study a disease or disorder. The public health department job is to conduct studies that are epidemiological in nature in order to prevent contagious disease from spreading. An epidemiologist is one who understands the rate/risk ratios, rate/risk differences, and measures the impact on the public.

Each epidemiologist deals in his own science and disciplines when he is taking these factors and measuring them. The discipline requires him to be able to select and use appropriate statistical methods in the analysis of simple data sets and apply these methods by computer using either STATA or EPI-INFO. He must also be able to understand and interpret output from statistical analyses carried out by computer, in relation to research and other questions asked. Then the epidemiologist must present findings based on statistical analysis in a clear concise manner.

The epidemiologist must be able to define a research problem and formulate a study hypothesis and objectives. He must choose an appropriate and ethical study design, plan field procedures, including sample selection, and the design of questionnaires and record forms. A time schedule for the conduct of the study is vital part. The need to prepare a budget is always important for this type of research. A detailed protocol that is of sufficient standard developed into a submission statement for a funding agency.

The epidemiologist must understand the basic statistical measures and concepts underlying the analysis of epidemiological data. He must perform analyses of data arising from epidemiological studies using appropriate computer software. He must be able to identify factors that suggest a disease has an infectious cause. He also must understand the factors determining the spatial, temporal and social distributions of communicable diseases. It is vital that the epidemiologist understand how to measure transmissibility of infections, design, and carry out, analyses, interpret and report an outbreak investigation report. It is of course very vital that the evaluation of vaccine efficacy be investigated.

The study of epidemiology and the use of an epidemiologist are vital for any nation's health. This is very important for it helps the nation prevent major breakouts of diseases. I would like to say our people do an excellent job in this field and their tasks are not always easy but always necessary. The American Heart Association feels that since heart failure is the number one killer of men and women in America today that our Public Health Department is not fulfilling their duties toward heart related diseases.

In the above description of what epidemiologist, duties are and why we have the study of epidemiology gives a better understanding the medical field problems concerning heart failure patients. The AHA has gathered as much information as possible thru magazines and articles and made a journal for the doctors to refer themselves too. That journal is piece meal at best, not complete and not adequate for the care and prevention of heart related problems. That is why we need an epidemiologist from our Public health Department to look at the situation.

# Heart Failure

Whenever cardiac conditions develop these conditions, weaken or damage your heart, which leads to heart failure. In a weakened condition, the heart over time can no longer keep up with even the normal demands placed on it. The ventricles may become stiff and not fill properly between beats. The heart ventricles stretch (dilate) to the point that the heart cannot pump blood efficiently throughout your body. The failing pump causes blood and fluid to back up throughout your circulatory system. The circulatory system consists of your lungs, legs, feet and ankles. The kidneys retain excess water and sodium. All this builds up is the congestive part of your heart failure. The lung congestion occurs only with left-sided heart failure with fluid backing up into the lungs. The most common cause of right sided heart failure is left sided heart failure.

When the fluid fills up the left side of the heart the pressure in the lungs passes to the right side of the heart, which then fails. The fluid then collects in the abdomen and lower extremities which all leads up to heart failure. Heart Failure develops quickly after a heart attack. The heart failure can also develop after years of high blood pressure or coronary artery disease. A defective valve may cause heart failure. A heart valve replacement in this case will prevent heart failure. A specialist normally does the surgical part, which is a cardiologist.

Many times people think that such things cause heart failure as smoking, being overweight or eating foods high in cholesterol and fat but there is a condition known as idiopathic dilated cardiomyopathy were the heart weakens without explanation. This condition will also cause you congestive heart failure if not properly taken seriously.

You might be suffering from if you have heart failure several conditions. These conditions can weaken your heart over time and be present without you being aware that you have the problem. The follow is a brief description of some conditions that affect the heart:

- The most common cause of heart failure is *Coronary Artery Disease*. A process called atherosclerosis, which is a build-up of fatty deposits in the arteries. This fatty build-up causes the arteries to narrow, a process called plaque, which leaves the heart chronically deprived of oxygen-rich blood and pumps less vigorously. A heart attack occurs if an unstable plaque detaches from the arteries and causes a blood clot; in turn it completely blocks the blood flow to an area of the heart muscle. This is one of the most common causes of heart failure.

- There are several other reasons that might cause heart failure but we shall discuss the next highest reason for now. High Blood Pressure (hypertension) is the force of blood pumped by your heart through your arteries. When your blood pressure is high then your heart has to work harder causing failure.

Take your cardiologists advice watch your weight and exercise, you're on the way to a heart healthy way of life.

# Congestive Heart

A congestive heart can be fatal without the proper treatments. That is why today organizations spend a lot of time and resources researching for cures and preventatives.

When you suffer from having a congestive heart then the heart is not able to maintain adequate circulation of blood in the tissues of the body or to pump out the venous blood returned to it by venous circulation. It is very important for all patients to understand what their heart is doing so they may take action to prevent any failure by the heart.

We do realize that you cannot see inside your chest and know what is going on but there are symptoms that will clue you into the fact that you are having some problems. All of a sudden, you notice that you have a shortness of breath whenever you try to walk or go up and down steps. This is one of the major signs of heart congestion.

All of a sudden, you realize that you tire easily and feel constantly tired even after a good nights rest. Fatigue and tiring is another signal that you should call your physician with concerns about your possibility of congestive heart problems. When you find the swelling of the feet, ankles, legs and occasionally the abdomen are constant and very discomforting then you should check with your doctor. Persistent coughing, raspy breathing or wheezing is another symptom of having a congestive heart.

"If you experience any of these symptoms, contact your doctor."

Suddenly you find that you are gaining weight and have no way of controlling this gain. When you diet but still find that you are gaining weight, perhaps the problem is with your heart. The fact that you are still gaining weight without any cause may have cause for alarm. This is a symptom of a congestive heart. Breathing can become rather difficult even when you are lying down. A cough or wheeze may also occur along with spitting up red sputum. These are all signals of a congestive heart and you should see your physician before it becomes congestive heart failure.

You are really into problems if you have chest pain feel palpitations of the heart and develop a fever do not hesitate go straight to the emergency room as this is a signal that your congestive heart failure is happening. You might have started out with some ankle swelling, feet swelling and leg swelling at that point I would immediately contact my physician. I am sure that at this point your physician will send you to a cardiologist. A cardiologist is a heart specialist.

A heart specialist can make suggestions that will help you maintain a healthy life style and provide you with the proper medical care. A proper diet is essential in having a healthy heart. Medicine has improved over the years and so has procedures that your cardiologist will advise you. Congestive heart problems need not become a situation of heart failure.

# What is CHF?

It's a terrifying moment for many patients: the moment when the doctor enters their hospital room and informs them they are suffering from Congestive Heart Failure (CHF). Many people do not know what congestive heart failure is or what it means for their life, and they ask themselves, "Is congestive heart failure the end of my world as I know it?"

Congestive heart failure occurs when for whatever reason the heart is unable to effectively pump the blood through the body. This usually occurs when the heart muscle is weak due to disease or stressed beyond its ability to function. Congestive heart failure is usually a secondary disease following another cardiac condition, primarily coronary artery disease, cardiomyopathies, myocarditis, valvular disease, or cardiac arrhythmias, with coronary artery disease carrying the poorest prognosis. It may also follow a myocardial infarction, renal failure, sepsis or severe anemia.

Each side of the heart has a different function, and therefore will have a slightly different effect on the body when it is unable to fulfill that function. If it is the left side of the heart that has failed accumulation of fluid in and around the lungs will cause the patient to experience difficulty breathing, and the kidneys will respond to the reduced blood in the circulation by retaining fluid as well. If it is the right side that fails the excess fluid accumulates in the venous system, giving the patient a generalized edema that becomes more severe as their condition deteriorates.

Dyspnea is the prevalent presenting symptom in congestive heart failure, although the severity will vary from patient to patient. Some will possess perfectly normal pulmonary function until under exertion, such as while exercising, walking up stairs or mowing their lawn; others will have so much fluid accumulated that simply rising from bed in the morning will prove difficult. These patients will also usually become easily fatigued due to a lack of oxygen to the tissues. Heart failure will also cause a condition known as pitting edema, in which the body retains fluid to the point that when pressure is applied to specific spot on the body the indentation remains (non-pitting edema is not caused by heart failure).

Treatment of congestive heart failure consists primarily of treating the symptoms. Vital signs should be taken regularly, and often diuretics will be prescribed to facilitate expulsion of accumulated fluid from the body. While in the hospital fluid intake and output will be measured very carefully. Patients will probably be placed in an upright position to assist in moving fluid from around the heart and lungs, given potassium supplements and prescribed bed rest for a period of time. BUN levels and serum creatinine, potassium, sodium, chloride and bicarbonate levels are monitored frequently by a physician.

There are several factors that contribute to congestive heart failure and, if diagnosed, should be treated and maintained. These include hypertension, anemia or poycythemia, endocrine disorders, malnutrition, drug or alcohol use and obesity. Therefore, it is very important that patients suffering from congestive heart failure pay particular attention to maintaining a healthy lifestyle. A doctor can aid in establishing the best diet and exercise plan with each individual to prevent placing undue stress on the heart and lungs.

While no said cure exists for congestive heart failure and the prognosis varies from case to case, by following a strict diet and exercise program, taking all prescribed medications regularly and maintaining a close relationship with their physicians many patients who suffer from heart failure can continue to lead a fairly normal life.

# Congestive Heart Failure

The human body is a magnificent machine that works in harmony with nature. The machinery needs proper care and sometimes parts replaced. Like the machine so the heart also needs help to prevent failure. The pump may not pump enough blood to meet your body's needs, which can lead into congestive heart failure. Many underlying conditions can cause congestive heart failure.

Over time and with the wear and tear of one's body the heart itself can develop such things as coronary artery disease or high blood pressure, which can lead to congestive heart failure. These things sap your strength leaving the heart with the inability to pump efficiently causing a break down. It is very important that you take care of yourself because these things while not reversible are preventable.

We have medicines that can treat the conditions you have improving your survival rate. These medications if taken properly can help control your blood pressure, cholesterol levels, and other things that might be affecting your heart. The field of medicine has come a very long way in providing medicines to prevent congestive heart failure.

The cardiologist, who is a heart specialist, can inform you about by-pass surgery or stents to help open up the flow of your blood through your veins. Many things are possible to prolong your life just ask your doctor for advise as to what you need. It is very possible for you to do things for yourself that will help in good heart health.

Congestive heart failure maybe prevented by changing your lifestyle. This does not always take a big change but some things in your life are controllable. First, look at your diet eat a heart healthy diet. Watch out for salt intake, fatty foods, and over indulgences as these can cause congestive heart failure. Many of us in today's world need to know how to manage stress overcome depression or simply improve the quality of our life. The problem of being overweight can lead to other problems such as coronary artery disease, high blood pressure, high cholesterol and diabetes. We need to keep these conditions under control in order to prevent congestive heart failure.

Managing stress becomes a stressful problem in itself for many people. While others enjoy the benefit of belonging to a gym or owning equipment that they use in their homes some of us do not have the time, money, or space to afford such luxury's. A person who sits daily in his office may feel the tensions building up to the point of no relief and farther some even go into a depressive condition. This is very bad for the heart we say that our heart is what feels our emotions like love, sadness, hate, excitement etc. still yet our heart suffers with stress and depression. Congestive heart failure one of the number one killers of men and women can be prevented. Prevention begins as they say at home with you taking care of your needs.

# CHF Diagnosis

While all cardiac conditions carry similar symptoms of chest pain and difficulty breathing, congestive heart failure generally presents with a very specific set of symptoms and lab results, giving doctors a very firm set of clues upon which to base a definite diagnosis.

Dyspnea, or difficulty breathing, coupled with severe pitting edema (when the body retains fluid to the point of holding the imprint of an object that is pressed into the skin for several minutes) are generally the first pieces of evidence pointing to congestive heart failure. Heart failure results in the heart not being able to efficiently pump blood throughout the body; as a result, fluid accumulates rather than being excreted and causes the body to swell as if it were a water balloon. Non-pitting edema, or fluid retention that does not hold an imprint, is not caused by heart failure and indicates that another diagnosis needs to be made. The patient may produce a frothy pink sputum when they cough.

In addition to the symptoms related to the fluid accumulation general weakness and malaise, particularly during times of physical exertion are frequent complaints of patients suffering from congestive heart failure, and should not be ignored. This is caused by a lack of nutrients and oxygen from the blood to the body tissues, and may result in permanent damage to the organs if they are left without these vital elements for a prolonged period of time. Anuria, or a lack of urination, is also evidential of heart failure as fluid accumulates in the tissues rather than being properly excreted. Patients may suffer from a changed mental status due to toxins accumulating in the body.

Once the physician suspects heart failure based on the physical evidence, blood samples will be sent to the laboratory. Beta-natriuretic peptide, or BNP, is an excellent screening tool in suspected cases of heart failure. This hormone is produced in greater quantities by the failing heart muscle as fluid levels rise, with a level between one hundred and five hundred pg/mg suggesting congestive heart failure and greater than five hundred being fairly diagnostic; however, an elevated BNP should not be considered to be sufficient evidence upon which to base a positive diagnosis, as conditions such as renal failure, ventricular strain, tumors or hypoxia can also cause BNP levels to rise. Arterial blood gases may be tested to determine the degree of hypoxemia. A decreased erythrocyte sedimentation rate, proteinuria (protein in the urine), and a mild azotemia (elevated blood urea level) can be seen in early to moderate disease. An increased serum creatinine, hyperbilirubinemia (increased bilirubin in the blood) and dilutional hyponatremia (decreased serum sodium levels) are evidence the patient is suffering from a more advanced case of heart failure.

Radiology will also wish to perform imaging studies to evaluate the condition of the heart. A chest x-ray will generally reveal cardiomegaly (enlargement of the heart) and pleural effusion (fluid around the heart). An echocardiogram may be performed to evaluate the internal structures of the heart to evaluate for any structural abnormalities, as in the case of mitral stenosis. This provides evidence to determine the underlying cause of congestive heart failure, particularly in suspected cases of valvular heart disease.

Physicians are like detectives, if you will. Once these tests have all been run they will gather these pieces of evidence together and put them together to form a fairly accurate picture of the patient's condition, allowing for an accurate diagnosis leading to proper treatment.

# New Therapies for Treatment of CHF

Heart disease is one of the deadliest killers in the world to date. Congestive heart failure, a condition found secondary to many major cardiac diseases, possesses its own high mortality rate. Fifty percent of those diagnosed with congestive heart failure will die within the five following years. Scientists and researchers are struggling to understand the exact mechanisms of the disease, and to find a cure.

Congestive heart failure results as the cells in the heart die or become non-functioning due to an event such as a myocardial infarction (a heart attack) or ischemic heart disease. Whatever the cause, the heart is subsequently unable to pump blood adequately throughout the body, resulting in the blood pooling in the organs and fluid building up in and around the lungs as sodium is unable to be properly excreted, causing the dyspnea that is the classic symptom of congestive heart failure.

Clinical research is targeted at both the treatment of the disease and the possibility of repairing the damaged cells in the heart. Current research is underway to test new medications that would assist in vasodilation, as well as a calcium inhibitor that would not result in the higher incidence of cardiac arrhythmia seen with the medications currently on the market.

In the age of natural medicine, the power of the mind has been invoked in clinical trials to use meditation and relaxation techniques to combat the stress on the heart that can be the breaking point for patients with heart failure. Stress has been shown to negatively affect the body's blood pressure, forcing the heart to work harder and placing an undue amount of pressure on an already weakened muscle. The theory lies in the belief that by learning to maintain a low level of mental stress the heart will be less stressed and therefore less likely to fail completely, and the patient can be given a better prognosis.

Alongside the return to natural, holistic methods of treatment is an incredible advancement in clinical technology that was not available twenty or thirty years ago. Scientists claim to have identified a set of altered genes that can make an individual more disposed to suffer from congestive heart failure and are using their current knowledge of genes and the benefits of gene therapy to attempt to reverse the effect. In addition, medications to clamp down on the genes' activities, such as beta blockers and alpha-2 agonists are already available and are being used in treatment programs.

Also being explored is the possibility of using stem cells, the body's pluripotent progenitors, to assist in reparation of the damaged heart tissue. Clinical trials showed that patients suffering from congestive heart failure responded very favorably to an injection of their own stem cells into the heart, although the exact means by which this causes improvement is as yet unknown. It is suspected that these cells either facilitate the growth of new vessels in the heart or act as beacon, attracting the body's own healing cells to the site of the damage and stimulating repair.

The possibility of actually growing healthy tissue from embryonic stem cells to be transplanted is also being explored, although the controversial nature of the use of embryonic stem cells due to the necessary destruction of the embryo makes this questionable in the foreseeable future. Scientists have determined that adult stem cells simply cannot provide an adequate number of new cells to meet the needs of patients who have suffered heart failure.

Heart failure is incredibly dangerous because the body cannot reproduce the dead tissue cells in the heart; however, with modern advancements it is the great hope of researchers everywhere to one day find a cure.

# Top Hospitals- Lower Mortality Rate

The American Heart Association did a new study concerning hospitals and their mortality rates. We now know that the top 5 percent in the United States have a 28% lower death rate than other hospitals in the nation. Health Grades is an independent health care ratings company released this information January 29th, 2010. They also found that patients who have surgery at the top-rated hospitals are about five percent less likely to suffer complications than patients at other hospitals are.

The Health Grade Company analyzed death and mortality rates for 26 procedures and diagnoses, including bypass surgery, angioplasty, stroke, and heart attack, at all 5,122 nonfederal hospitals. The top hospitals reduced their death rate by an average of 11.7 percent and reduced post-surgical complication rates by 3.4 percent. The study author claimed that if all U.S. hospitals had the same quality of care as the top hospitals, 158,264 lives would have been saved and 12,409 major complications avoided. Unfortunately, there is a gap in the quality of care provided by high quality hospitals and other hospitals in the United States, according to Health Grades.

In order to qualify for the Health Grades list, hospitals were required to meet minimum thresholds in terms of patient volumes, quality ratings and the range of services provided.

In the top 5% of hospitals that deal with heart, patients there are 229 in the nation today. The hospitals are located

32

all around the nation and keep a high standard of performance.

The Christ Hospital located in Cincinnati, Ohio ranked number one in cardiovascular care is affiliated with several other hospitals in the area that are accredited as being in the top 100 of the 5% heart hospitals.

One of the most distinguished top cited heart hospitals and medical centers is the Robert Wood Johnson's University Hospital. This hospital has earned significant national recognition for clinical quality and patient safety. This hospital is the principal teaching hospital of the University of Medicine in the state of New Jersey. It is a very demanding position to be the one is who teach others how to take care of heart patients.

The Dayton Heart Hospital focus on patient care and fighting any problems that deals with heart problems. Each year heart disease kills more people than any other disease. Patients want new and better ways of healing. The physicians, community leaders, and others want to reduce the impact of heart disease has on society.

Spectrum Hospital in Grand Rapids, Michigan has updated its heart wing, is now one of the leading hospitals for open-heart surgery, and transplants. The staff at Spectrum Hospital is very sensitive to patient needs and stress levels and tries to help in any manner possible. When a patient leaves the hospital, the care does not stop at that point. They provide in home nurses that visit the patient on a daily basis to make sure that they are coming along very well. Therapy is a part of the patient care after a month or so when the patient feels they are ready. The patient then goes to the therapy wing and a professional helps lead in proper therapy techniques. The hospital also provides a dietician who helps with your diet plan. The care provided is necessary for complete recovery.

# Patients' Needs for a Healthy Heart

The American College of Cardiology had a meeting to discuss a number of controversial findings on how to treat a patient with congestive heart failure. Not every person is a like therefore; a treatment for one Patient may not work on another one. This has left many Patients scratching their heads over the proper treatment for their cardiovascular condition. The experts have admitted that what works for one heart patient may not work for another one.

There was a study of over 2,300 patients where angioplasty-vs-drug therapy comparison proved the same. The result was that no differences in death, nonfatal heart attacks, strokes or hospitalization between patients with "stable" heart disease treated with medication alone vs. those who got drugs plus angioplasty and stenting.

A physician realizes that you as a patient know your own body and know your own needs such as diets and exercise. A Patients treatment by the medical field solely based accordingly to their needs and accessibility of medical procedures. Each patient should have the right to know what his care will be and what he can do to help prevent congestive heart failure. The patient should plan to make for him or herself a plan of action that will have a healthy lifestyle. Start with diet and exercise the two most important things in your life to improve upon in order to have a healthy heart.

The Patient still has rights over their own body as to the type of treatment and care they want to receive. The Patient should make a list of what they feel in order to discuss with the doctor the symptoms that they are suffering. This will help your doctor in diagnosis of your case and determine the treatment and care that is best for you. You should be able to confer with your physician on any type of treatment recommended and ask for a second opinion if you are not sure about what the procedures recommended for you are right. You can start your own program to help with your condition if you find that congestive heart failure is just around the corner or you already show symptoms.

First, look at your weight. Are you overweight? Do you need a diet? You know the answers to these questions all too well. A diet plan should fit your physical needs, which will help you lose weight and keep the weight off as well. You do not have to join a group or special buy your food in order to go on a diet. There are adequate diets plans available free on the internet. You should check with your physician before you attempt a diet plan. The next thing that you can do is exercise to help lose weight and relieve stress. You can become your own Patient keep track of your vitals, weight loss and any other important information about yourself. A Patient has power to control the way that they live their life.

# Combat Congestive Heart Failure

Congestive heart failure is an insidious opponent, possessing a slow onset that results in a patient often not even noticing they are having symptoms. Over time the patient will suffer from worsening dyspnea and edema that will eventually drive them to seek treatment, where they will discover that for whatever reason their heart is no longer able to function properly.

Heart failure occurs when the cells of the heart tissue are either destroyed or made non-functional due to another cardiac event, often secondary to ischemic heart disease or coronary artery disease. As a result, the heart is no longer able to pump the blood throughout the body properly; instead the blood pools, resulting in fluids being retained rather than excreted properly and oxygen starved organs being unable to function. The death of these cells is critical because, like brain cells, once the cells of the heart die the body is unable to reproduce them and restore full function to the heart. *Congestive heart failure carries with it a high mortality rate, with over fifty percent of its victims dying within five years of being diagnosed.* Doctors and researchers are able to use modern advancements in medicine to make the patient more comfortable and, in many cases, to provide them with a more favorable prognosis.

Many patients do not even discover that they have suffered heart failure until they are brought into the Emergency Department of their local hospital complaining of chest pain and difficulty breathing. Doctors will stabilize them there, giving them supplemental oxygen and beginning a course of medicinal treatment that will carry them out of the hospital.

Modern science has provided physicians with a wide array of methods with which to combat the damage done by congestive heart failure. Once oxygen is returned to an acceptable level a physician will usually administer a diuretic to stimulate the renal system to pull fluid out of circulation, relieving the edema and taking a great of stress off of the lungs, heart and other organs. This will also usually be accompanied by supplemental potassium, as the renal system will remove potassium along with the excess fluid and hypokalemia carries with it its own hazards.

A great deal of attention in the field of medicine has been focused on the body's production of angiotensin II as it aggravates congestive heart failure. Angiotensin II is a substance produced by the body which raises blood pressure and causes the blood vessels to constrict, thereby forcing the heart to work much harder to pump blood throughout the body. An ACE inhibitor will often be administered to prevent the body from making angiotensin II, and an angiotensin receptor blocker is available to those who do not respond as desired to the ACE inhibitor. Many patients with heart problems are given nitroglycerin for this reason.

Along with medicine, research into the field of congestive heart failure is ongoing. The speculated use of stem cells, particularly embryonic stem cells, has opened a whole field of debate for possible treatment of heart failure in the science community. Patients with congestive heart failure were given some of their own stem cells in the heart via injection, and all reacted favorably. Scientists are unsure as to whether this is because the stem cells aid the body in growing new vessels or simply act as a lighthouse for the body's natural healing mechanisms, drawing other cells to the site of the damage. Whichever the case may be, stem cells present a fascinating opportunity to finally find a means by which to restore heart function to patients who have suffered heart failure.

Modern science is providing a whole new world of treatment options to patients with congestive heart failure, and researchers are making new discoveries all the time. It is the hope of all of those in the medical field that one day heart failure will be another disease medicine has the answer to.

# Saving the Heart

There is no cure for congestive heart failure, but there are things that you can do to help prolong your life and protect your heart from farther damage. Treatment is a matter of changing your lifestyle and drug therapy, which will change your quality of life. The medical field improvement over the past twenty years has grown in leaps and bounds. Lifestyle changes are the same quit smoking, losing excess weight, drinking less alcohol, and eating healthy low saturated fat and low salt foods. Then do not forget to exercise which is helpful for most patients. This is good advice that is a key to preventing heart failure but the most important is the medical. This is where your physician is very important; do not attempt to try to prescribe your own medicines. The physician is well equipped to provide you with the proper medical treatment.

The heart like other parts of our bodies can malfunction in different ways. That is why we should trust the cardiologist, a specialist in the medical field. One of the most common medicines prescribed for patients is a beta-blocker. The beta-blocker reduces the heart rate and output of blood by counteracting a hormone called noradrenalin. While this drug can prevent heart failure, it is not recommended for anyone with severe heart failure.

Patients who suffer from fluid retention and/or high blood pressure the medical field suggests that a diuretic will help compensate but some of the side effects is loss of potassium, weakness, muscle cramps, and joint pains. Let your doctor know right away if you feel any ill effects from the diuretic.

This is just an example of some drugs used by the medical field that can help prevent heart failure. There are other treatments that the medical field uses are just as valuable.

Congestive heart failure can become quiet extreme that is why the medical field has been experimenting with heart transplants and mechanical pumps, which are attached to the heart. There is another experimental procedure for severe heart failure, which is available at a few U.S. medical centers. This procedure, called cardiomyoplasty, involves detaching one end of a muscle in the back, wrapping it around the heart, and then suturing the muscle to the heart. An implanted electric stimulator causes the back muscle to contract and pump blood from the heart.

The medical field has also another surgical procedure called mitral valve repair may help extend and improve the lives of people with congestive heart failure. This procedure aims to correct leaky valves resulting from cardiomyopathy, or heart muscle disease, by surgically inserting a flexible annuloplasty ring at the mitral valve opening.

The medical field has made great strides in medicines and in surgical procedures that greatly increase the quality of life, we have. The medical field has experimented with such things as healthy heart diets and specialized exercises that can only help to improve quality of life. Now it is up to you it is your heart!

# Living With Heart Failure

Heart failure, as well as all the risks that accompany it, can be a terrifying prospect for any man, woman or child. The impact of a heart, the body's central tool for survival, no longer functioning may seem like the beginning of the end. The good news is, by establishing an effective treatment plan with your cardiologist the prognosis, and the chances for you to lead a normal life, increase exponentially.

Heart failure occurs when the heart can no longer efficiently pump blood throughout the body. The blood pools, and while organs are deprived of vital, life giving oxygen and nutrients the excess sodium that would normally be excreted in the urine builds up in the tissues, resulting in fluid retention that leads to organ stress and the dyspnea that is so common in cases of congestive heart failure. Left untreated, the oxygen deprived organs will eventually cease to function and the patient will die.

Fortunately, there are now many ways to combat the mortality factor associated with heart failure. Doctors can prescribe medications to facilitate the flow of blood through the body and take some of the pressure off the heart; blood thinners can decrease the chances of clots forming in the veins. Aside from medicinal means, there are many factors that may be altered in your lifestyle to impact the prognosis of your disease.

It is essential that the body be given sufficient time to rest in a day. While at rest the heart can more easily pump blood throughout the body; just as you would rest an injured leg when it began to pain you, you should rest your heart as well. On the flip side, it is important to establish a daily exercise routine. It doesn't have to be three hours of aerobics; a half hour walk every day would have a greater impact on your physical being than nothing. Consult with your physician to find the plan that works best for your individual circumstances.

Along with an exercise plan you should work with your doctor to find the best diet plan for you. In most cases a low sodium diet is recommended to help reduce fluid retention. Diuretics can greatly affect the levels of potassium in the body causing hypokalemia, which can lead to muscle weakness, paralysis and a fatal cardiac arrhythmia; therefore, very often if you have been given a diuretic to take daily a potassium supplement will also be prescribed.

Nicotine can create a serious problem for patients with heart failure. It increases the heart rate and blood pressure while having a negative impact on the oxygen level in the blood. All of these things cause the heart to work harder. It is strongly recommended that if you have been diagnosed with heart failure you quit smoking completely.

Hand in hand with smoking are the inherent dangers associated with contracting a case of pneumonia or flu. If you are able you should receive an annual flu shot, as well as the one time dose of pneumococcal vaccine. This will provide some level of protection against pneumococci bacteria, the major cause of bacterial pneumonia. Pneumonia is a problem for the same reasons as smoking; the decreased oxygen levels in the blood cause the heart to work harder in an attempt to compensate and get oxygen to the organs and tissues. If possible, avoid crowded areas during cold and flu season, and stay away from people you know are sick.

Amazingly, something as simple as the clothes you wear can impact your condition if you have suffered heart failure. Tight clothing can cause blood clots and restrict blood flow to the extremities. In addition, in cases of extreme temperature your clothes should be weather appropriate; if the body has to work to maintain its temperature the heart will have to work that much harder.

Sexual relations can usually be continued as before; however, they should occur in as peaceful an environment as possible to prevent undue stress. If your condition is severe it is important that you discuss this with your physician; it may be necessary to forego sexual relations for a time in favor of other, less stressful shows of affection.

Each of these steps will help you continue to live much as you did before being diagnosed. Heart failure will inevitably impact your life; it is entirely up to you how much.

# Current Research on CHF

Medical research is a never ending fount of information, and its sources are vast. Unfortunately, it may be very difficult for a layman not associated with the medical field to find up to date information pertaining to his disease and treatment options. While doctors are constantly attending conferences as part of their continuing education curriculum, the average Joe is left to sort through a variety of sources in an attempt to find information that is not obsolete. The best choice for this patient is to continue his research in one of the many scientific research journals published.

While a specific journal pertaining solely to the topic of congestive heart failure may not be available, there are a seemingly infinite number of research journals being published that pertain to medical issues (there are research journals published for any field in which there is someone doing research). These are available in both a virtual format or in a hard copy. If a research source is found that a patient particularly favors they can purchase a subscription, which will allow them to receive new issues of the journal as they are released. When researching a specific topic or disease purchasing a subscription to just one source may not be the action of choice. Often a variety of articles pertaining to a specific topic can be found in multiple journals, and it is often more beneficial to read more than one. Libraries will often carry a subscription to several periodicals, and many will publish an edition over the internet. A portion of the journals that can be found online allow readers full access without a subscription.

Scientific journals publish cutting edge research, giving the average person a chance to read about advances in medicine and technology that are occurring in every field. It was a scientific journal that first published the information about stem cell research that sparked a controversy across the nation, and these same stem cells are now considered one of the best chances for providing long term relief for patients suffering from heart failure. Through scientific journals the reader is taken through laboratories around the world and exposed to ideas and theories of some of the planet's greatest minds.

When searching for a research journal from which to learn it is important to ascertain that it is, in fact, a reputable source. Research journals publish both theory and fact, and it is essential that the two be differentiated. A publication with a reputation of publishing theories as facts should be avoided. If a patient is unfamiliar with the world of science it would probably be helpful for them to seek the aid of their physician in finding a factual source of information which publishes only peer reviewed articles and up to date research.

It is important to remember that the articles written in scientific journals are written by health professionals for health professionals, and may be very difficult for a person uneducated in anatomy and medical terminology to understand; however, when armed with a dictionary and a physician to consult with scientific journals are an endless source of information.

# Peer Review in Medical Research

When seeking information on the latest updates in the field of medicine the best place to look is in a peer reviewed scientific journal. It is essential that a journal be peer reviewed to ensure that information is as accurate and up to date as possible.

Many publications do not utilize the process of peer review for its articles. Many common periodicals are examples of this. Magazines such as Cosmo, Good Housekeeping, and Time magazine are examples of this. It is up to an editor to decide whether or not to make an article available for public consumption. The flaw in this system can be found in the simple fact that no one is able to know everything about everything. Editors can make mistakes based on their own lack of knowledge. In addition, articles written based upon personal opinion, unfounded statements or biased research may be printed, which is fine if the periodical is searching for an opinion but not so valued when the reader is searching for cold, hard fact. By using peer review, much of this possibility is eliminated.

The process of peer review (or refereeing, as it is also known as in the scientific community) is very simple. All articles written concerning research projects to be published will be submitted to the editor of the journal in question. Copies of the article are then distributed to two or three experts in the field of which the article is written (for example, an article concerning congestive heart failure would be submitted to several experts in the field of cardiology). These professionals (the author's "peers") will then evaluate the article for accuracy, quality and relevance to the journal the author wishes it to be published in and submit their evaluation to the editor of the article in question. In this way a great pool of knowledge is being combined to decide if an article is fit for publication.

In the past reviewers have normally retained anonymity, both to the author whose work they have reviewed and the general public, preventing an author from launching a personal vendetta against a specific reviewer; however, in some instances editors have allowed an author to make a rebuttal to a reviewer who had criticized their work, particularly if an article received mixed reviews. This system is gradually changing, as cries for accountability are becoming heard. The Journal of Interactive Media in Education was among the first to utilize an open peer review system, by which reviewers names are made public and they may be held accountable for their statements.

Peer reviewed journals are generally easily distinguished from other periodicals. They present a much more sedate appearance and utilize a great deal of technical language, and all sources will be cited. Topics will focus on scientific research rather than general events, and are quite obviously focused towards fellow professionals in the field rather than the average reader. If they are unsure as to whether a publication has been peer reviewed a number of sources are available for scholars which provide a listing of peer reviewed journals across the country.

# Treatment of Congestive Heart Failure

Congestive heart failure is precisely what it sounds like; it is a failure of the heart to properly function, and its effects on the body can be devastating. Physicians do their best to treat the symptoms and give the patient the best prognosis possible; however, no true cure for congestive heart failure currently exists.

Heart failure occurs when the heart is unable to properly pump blood throughout the body; as a result, rather than distributing nutrients and oxygen to the tissues and then excreting the excess fluid into the urine the blood pools. This results in either a systemic or localized edema as fluid builds up in the veins and organs, causing swelling of the extremities as well as the organs themselves (this fluid accumulation is responsible for an excessive amount of stress on the heart as fluid accumulates in the pleural cavity as well as the dyspnea, or difficulty breathing, often symptomatic of heart failure). The swelling and lack of oxygen and nutrients will result in permanent damage to the organs if left untreated, providing a very poor prognosis for the patient.

The first stage of treatment generally consists of the administration of extra oxygen to attempt to return the oxygen levels in the tissues to normal. Once oxygen has been administered and a pulse oximeter reveals blood oxygen levels to be acceptable the focus will shift to attempting to treat the fluid build-up in the body. Diuretics will be administered to assist the excess fluid on its path out of the body via the urinary tract, and nitrates are administered to cause the vessels to dilate, allowing blood to flow more freely without the heart having to work quite as hard. Treatment with diuretics is often accompanied by supplemental potassium, as the body will excrete potassium in the urine and long term hypokalemia may result in muscle weakness or paralysis, as well as an increased risk of fatal cardiac arrhythmia.

Patients will often be sent home from the hospital with diuretics, as well as a medication known as an ACE inhibitor (an angiotensin-converting enzyme inhibitor) which prevents the body from creating angiotensin, a substance which raises blood pressure and causes the blood vessels to constrict. An angiotensin II receptor blocker may also be administered if the patient continues to produce angiotensin. Patients may also be treated with vasodilators other than ACE inhibitors, particularly if they have responded poorly to treatments with ACE inhibitors in the past. Nitroglycerin is a common example of this type of medication.

Digitalis, or Digoxin, may be prescribed to strengthen the force of the heart's contractions, aiding it to push blood throughout the body. Treatment with a beta blocker is also beneficial in cases of heart failure, preventing the heart from beating more rapidly in an attempt to compensate for the poor movement of the blood in the body and placing more stress on the weakened muscle.

Blood thinners are used to prevent the formation of clots in the body that may be caused by the decreased movement of the blood in the vessels. Coumadin and heparin are the most commonly prescribed blood thinners in use today; however, due to an increased risk of bleeding patients taking these medications should undergo coagulation testing regularly.

Lifestyle changes are just as important as medications in the long term treatment of heart failure. Patients should consult with their doctor to establish an appropriate (low sodium) diet and exercise program, and should do at least some moderate exercise daily. Equally important is taking sufficient time to rest every day. The heart pumps more easily when the body is at rest, which is vital to an already overstressed muscle. The nicotine from cigarettes causes an increase in heart rate, blood pressure, and the tendency for clumping in the blood vessels; patients with heart failure should abstain from smoking. Flu or pneumonia can be very difficult for hearts that are failing as they attempt to compensate for the lack of oxygen in the bloodstream being carried to the organs. It is very important that patients receive an annual influenza vaccine, as well as a dose of the pneumococcal vaccine, which will protect them from the pneumococcal bacteria that cause over eighty percent of cases of bacterial pneumonia. Wearing non-constrictive clothing will assist in preventing blood clots and facilitating blood flow to the extremities, and in cases of extremely warm or extremely cold temperatures it is important that the patient take all precautions necessary to keep the body at an appropriate temperature..

Researchers are still seeking to find a cure for congestive heart failure; however, until that day comes it is extremely important that patients suffering from heart failure follow the treatment plan outlined by their physician. With careful attention to maintaining their condition, the prognosis associated with heart failure increases dramatically.

# Translational Research

In nature every action spawns a separate and equal reaction. In the field of medicine, the reaction may not always be equal to the action. The performance of a particular treatment in the lab on test animals may not be the same as would be seen in a human subject; this is where the field of translational research comes in.

Translational research takes research from the laboratory to the patient's bedside. This can be done in several forms. In its earliest stages a treatment will undergo controlled clinical trials with a voluntary group of test subjects. If these small, controlled tests meet the acceptable range of success the treatment is then taken to research hospitals such as St. Jude's or Children's Hospital of Boston. Here patients are given the opportunity to experience new methods of control and treatment of a disease with the understanding that it is still considered highly experimental; however, for many these treatments represent a chance for a cure that previously as out of reach for them as the moon.

Congestive heart failure is, at the moment, an incurable event, occurring when for whatever reason the cells of the heart muscle are destroyed and the heart can no longer adequately pump blood throughout the body. Once the cells in the heart tissue are non-functional the body is unable to replace them, making it impossible for the heart to regain full heart function on its own. The current mortality rate is high, and over fifty percent of patients with congestive heart failure will die within five years of being diagnosed. There are many treatment options currently being considered for congestive heart failure, however, and a number of new technologies being tested daily. For example, Montefiore Medical Center in New York City is currently doing clinical trials on a drug known as Lovosimendan, a calcium sensitizer that does not trigger cardiac arrhythmia, and research into the possibility of using stem cells to re-grow cardiac tissue is ongoing.

For a patient to take advantage of these options they should discuss the possibility of being a subject for clinical testing with their physician to see if they would be a good candidate, then allow the physician to make a recommendation on a course of action from there. It may be suggested that the patient contact a research facility or the physician may suggest their name for a clinical trial they know is occurring soon. If the patient lives in an area with a research hospital nearby, chances are there will be an opportunity for them to benefit from the hospital's policy on translational research.

It should be understood that translational research is precisely what it sounds like; research. Scientists and doctors are often still learning about the treatment and its effect on the human body, and there is always a possibility that it will be unsuccessful or carry with it many hazardous side effects. These courses of treatments are unknowns to physician and researcher alike. For patients who have run out of options, however, even the possibility of a negative effect cannot stifle what the opportunity to be part of a translational research project provides: hope.

# Stem Cells Use in Congestive Heart Failure

Heart failure is a devastating blow to the body system and despite the best efforts of clinicians and researchers often results in permanent organ damage and eventual death. Researchers are fighting to put a stop to the high mortality rate of congestive heart failure, and believe stem cells may be the way to do it.

The possible uses for stem cells have made it a highly published topic in medical journals today. Stem cells are the precursors to every cell in the body, and are primarily produced in the bone marrow in adults. During times of crisis, such as when a patient suffers from leukemia, the spleen and other organs that possessed stem cells during fetal development will take over production. This is the body's way of maintaining proper cell balances and replenishing itself as old cells die. For example, red blood cells in the circulation only have a lifespan of approximately four months; during that time the hematopoietic stem cells in the bone marrow are continuously producing new rubriblasts, the precursor cells that will over time become mature erythrocytes.

There are several forms of stem cells; for the sake of research scientists are currently focusing on the embryonic and adult varieties. Embryonic stem cells come from a blastocyst, a four to five day old human embryo. During gestation these pluripotent cells will divide and multiply, forming the body and internal organs of the fetus. Embryonic stem cells are highly valued for research for several reasons; they are able to provide large numbers of replenishing cells and have no limitations on what form of cells they can become. The use of embryonic stem cells is highly controversial, however, due to the fact that collection often requires the destruction of the embryo.

There are several methods that have been published in research journals regarding the application of stem cells in the treatment of congestive heart failure. Congestive heart failure results when cells in the heart are dysfunctional or destroyed and the heart is unable to properly pump blood throughout the body. Some patients are able to be treated using mechanical aids or transplant, but this is not always the case. Several years ago a group of patients with no other available options for treatment agreed to be part of a test study regarding stem cells. Autologous stem cells were removed from the marrow and injected into the failing heart tissue through the chest wall. Patients who received this treatment showed marked improvement, presumably as a result of stem cell action. The precise means by which this occurs is still unknown; however, research scientists speculate that the stem cell is either growing new vessels or acting as a beacon to bring other cells in to repair the damaged tissue.

Another possibility regarding stem cells is the growth of tissue for transplant. Hearts available for an organ transplant are not as easily obtained as physicians would desire, and there are often waiting lists years long for every available organ. Stem cells grow readily in a laboratory environment, and if unstimulated to differentiate will reproduce pluripotent daughter cells. This results in a tissue that will essentially adapt to whatever environment it is placed in. Research scientists speculate that with the proper environment essentially grow heart tissue and transplant it to the patient who has suffered heart failure, replacing the dead and damaged tissues with live, vital tissue. This procedure would allow the heart to function more easily and hopefully give the patient a better chance for survival.

With current treatment the prognosis for sufferers of congestive heart failure is grim. At least fifty percent will die within five years of being diagnosed, and those who are not victims of this mortality rate will feel the effects of their heart failure for the rest of their lives. Stem cell research represents a chance for those patients to beat these odds.

# Genes Contribute to and Cure Congestive Heart Failure

It is common knowledge that heart failure follows another severe form of heart damage; however, until now scientists and doctors have had no way to identify those at risk. New research into genes and gene therapy has made them a potential weapon in the fight against heart failure.

Scientists have made several discoveries regarding the role of genes in the detection and treatment of heart failure. Several years ago it was discovered that a small percentage of patients who had suffered heart failure possessed a defect in the gene that allows the body to detect stress signals; in essence, the heart does not know that it is working too hard and is unable to adjust. This percentage may seem insignificant; however, the gene mutation was not present in any of the healthy patients examined. Researchers stress that this is a susceptibility factor, not a cause of congestive heart failure; however, it may be the breaking point when determining if a heart suffering from other disease will fail. Detection of this mutation may allow doctors to identify and treat patients at risk prior to their heart failing rather than after.

This defect is found in the ATP-sensitive potassium channels and is caused by a genetic mutation. The potassium channel regulates potassium and calcium levels in the body. While the heart must have calcium to function, an excess of calcium leads to damage. This is the reason calcium blockers are often given to patients with congestive heart failure. Fortunately, medications to open the potassium channel already exist.

In addition, a defect of the delta-sarcoglycan gene has been seen in hamsters with muscular dystrophy and cardiomyopathy. This gene is the cytoskeleton of muscle fibers, and successful transplant of a normal human delta-sarcoglycan gene has been shown to cause a tremendous improvement in these animals. This is noteworthy because current transplant attempts require open heart surgery. This type of gene transplant is carried on a virus, eliminating the need for surgery.

Scientists had been a bit concerned with using this method of gene therapy due to the need for a systemic effect. There was also some concern that the body's natural immune system would eliminate the virus of its own accord prior to successful delivery of the gene; however, they believe they have found the best form of virus to successfully slip past the body's defenses. When transplanting the delta-sarcoglycan gene researchers used a type eight adeno-associated virus, piggybacking the corrective gene onto it as it was inserted into the body. This allowed the gene to be carried to all areas of the body in animals with muscular dystrophy without being destroyed by the body's own natural immunity.

Gene therapy is still highly experimental, and researchers are unsure yet of the role it will play in the conquest of heart failure; however, this represents a technology that was unavailable thirty years ago. Continuing advancements in technology and medicine's knowledge of the body's building blocks may one day unlock the mysteries to the cure of this deadly disease.

# Continuing Medical Education

While physicians spend many, many years in school prior to receiving their MD, it is impossible for them to learn everything there is to know. The medical field is simply too vast, and it is constantly in motion; therefore, it is important that every physician complete continuing medical education.

Continuing medical education (CME) allows a physician to stay abreast of new discoveries, treatments, and other advancements in their chosen field. What worked thirty years ago is not usually the method of choice for today's physicians, and clinicians who do not complete these continuing education credits may often be placing their patients at risk because of a lack of knowledge of treatments that have been deemed ineffective or hazardous. Unfortunately, often when a physician is wrong it is the patient's life that pays the price.

Due to this, every physician is required to complete a minimum number of CME credits every year; however, they are certainly not required stopping once that number is met. This does not necessarily mean returning to school, although this is certainly an option; however, for most physicians caring for their patients leaves them little time for the heavy workload of a secondary education institution. Many other more convenient options are available to them.

A cross the nation hundreds of thousands of medical conventions, symposiums, workshops and conferences are available to healthcare professionals, covering topics from new surgical techniques to treat collapsed heart valves to the use of stem cells to treat congestive heart failure; all cutting edge technology not yet taught in the classroom. These often take place over the course of a weekend, often last more than one day and are held in various locations, so physicians from any location in the country may attend at their discretion.

In many rural areas there is only one doctor available, often with no one to see to their patients when they are unavailable. These are the physicians who are still on call twenty four hours a day, make their own hospital rounds and see patients from birth to death for everything from a toothache to a heart attack. Needless to say they are often unable to get away from their practice to attend weekend workshops. Another option is available for them so they can continue to provide their patients with around the clock care. The internet has opened up a whole new world to the field of continuing education. Many organizations, such as the American Medical Association (AMA) and the American Association for Continuing Medical Education (AACME) offer resources online for healthcare workers to complete their continuing medical education credits. Here clinicians will have the opportunity to complete coursework online, view online conferences and use the teleweb to attend lectures and symposiums.

These CME resources may be found free of charge or for a small fee per credit hour, depending on the situation;

however, this is infinitely less expensive (and time consuming) than returning to a college or university, and offer greater benefits because attendees are able to stay apprised of new research and untried methods that are not taught to students.

It is true that no one ever stops learning, and this is especially true in the medical field. Continuing medical education allows clinicians to stay on top of their field and provide the best, most advanced care options available to their patients.

# Enjoy the Highest Quality of Life Possible With CHF

There is no doubt about it, cardiac complications can impact every corner of life, forcing patients to forego activities they previously enjoyed and causing them to feel as though they have sacrificed their life to save it. There are, however, many steps patients can take to allow them to enjoy life even after having been diagnosed with heart failure.

Congestive heart failure occurs when the cells of the heart are unable to constrict properly and pump blood through the body. This results in edema throughout the body, particularly in and around the lungs and is the cause of the dyspnea that is typical of heart failure. To counteract this, patients should take any diuretics prescribed by their doctor and maintain a low sodium diet, allowing the excess fluid to leave through the renal system and making it easier for the patient to breathe. Daily exercise is important; it is not necessary that it be vigorous, patients should consult with their physician prior to embarking on an exercise regime to ensure that they will not be taxing their heart unnecessarily. It is possible that if a patient has previously enjoyed activities that put a great deal of strain on the heart they will find it necessary to restrict themselves to less stressful endeavors; however, with the proper precautions many physical activities are still permitted.

The heart pumps blood more easily when the body is at rest; therefore, it is essential that patients with heart failure schedule time daily to rest. They may sit and read or watch television, take a nap or meditate; any activity that allows the body time to recharge. Meditation is being considered as a possible method of treatment for patients suffering from heart failure; meditation causes the heart to beat slower, blood pressure to normalize, the muscles to use oxygen more efficiently and the body to produce less adrenaline. All of these factors make it easier for the heart to function.

Any patient suffering from heart failure should abstain from smoking. Inhaling nicotine causes the body's blood pressure and heart rate to increase, less oxygen to reach the muscles and an increased clumping and stickiness in blood vessels that may impede blood flow. All of these factors cause the heart to beat harder in an attempt to compensate, placing more stress on an already weak heart.

Patients should also avoid flu and pneumonia as much as possible, avoiding crowded areas during cold and flu season and receiving both an annual influenza vaccination and at least one dose of the pneumococcal vaccine (this will provide some protection against pneumococcal bacteria, the most common cause of bacterial pneumonia). The decreased oxygen in the blood resulting from either flu or pneumonia will result in the heart pumping harder in an attempt to compensate.

Everything in their life affects a patient's well-being when they are suffering from congestive heart failure, right down to their clothing. These patients should avoid restrictive clothing and stockings as much as possible, as these items present an increased risk for clotting and a blockage of blood to the extremities. They should also avoid temperature extremes as much as possible and dress appropriately for the weather; the body must work much harder to maintain temperature when it is either extremely hot or extremely cold.

The most beneficial thing that patients suffering from heart failure can do to allow them to enjoy their life is to enjoy their life. The negative effects of stress on the heart are well documented, and patients who live a stress free existence create a much better environment for their heart than those who are unhappy or overworked. So by maintaining a positive mental state, patients are able to help themselves both emotionally and physically.

# Cardiac Professionals

In a field that is constantly shifting and changing, where researchers are finding new information almost daily and new diseases and symptoms are discovered with each patient it is very important for doctors and nurses to stay abreast of changes in the field. They do this through a variety of means, one of which is continuing education.

A cardiologist can spend twelve years or more in school prior to receiving their degree between undergrad school, medical school, residency, then additional coursework and residency to specialize. It may seem ludicrous to have to return to school after that period of time; after all, after ten years wouldn't they know all there is to know? The answer is no. The medical field is constantly open to new opportunities and knowledge; a cardiologist who graduated medical school thirty years would not have learned many of the new treatment and surgical options that are available today. They simply did not have the resources or technology then that they do now. Enter the field of continuing education.

Every clinician is required to complete a set number of continuing education credits on a regular basis, and to update these credits regularly. These credits do not have to be done by returning to an academic setting; most physicians would not have time to treat their patients and still take classes. Every year hundreds of symposiums, conferences and workshops are held throughout the world on a variety of topics. These each provide an established number of continuing education credits, and most clinicians will have to attend several of these to fulfill their continuing education requirement. Here cardiac professionals can learn about new techniques to treat a variety of diseases, such as the ongoing interest in using stem cells to strengthen the heart of patients with congestive heart failure, or the benefits of the newly released angiotensin II receptor blocker drugs. In this manner they are able to follow all of the advances in the field without having to abandon their practice and return to school.

The internet has also opened up a wonderful opportunity for health care professionals to complete their continuing education credits from the comfort of their homes. Many organizations offer online continuing education to healthcare professionals. They may complete coursework, watch online conferences, and virtually attend lectures. This is often the method of choice for physicians in rural areas who find it difficult to attend conferences due to their distance and the lack of other physicians to see their patients in their absence.

These continuing education credits may be available at no cost, or a reduced cost per credit hour, to physicians and group members. Continuing education is very important to healthcare professionals. A lack of continuing education will result in a clinician not being kept abreast of changes in the field, both positive and negative, and being unaware of which treatments have now been ruled ineffective or even hazardous. This will lead to being unable to properly treat their patients, and possibly endangering their lives in the process.